ESSENTIAL OIL SURVIVAL

*A QUICK REFERENCE GUIDE TO TREATING
COMMON AILMENTS NATURALLY*

By

JACK PENTAL

I0412538

Copyright © 2015

"*And by the river upon the bank thereof, on this side and on that side, shall grow all trees for meat, whose leaf shall not fade, neither shall the fruit thereof be consumed: it shall bring forth new fruit according to his months, because their waters they issued out of the sanctuary: and the fruit thereof shall be for meat, and the leaf thereof for medicine.*" ~ Ezekiel 47:12 - KJV

TABLE OF CONTENTS

Table of Contents

Legal Notes

AILMENTS

- Conjunctivitis - 30
- Constipation - 31
- Coughing - 32
- Diarrhea - 33
- Diverticulitis - 34
- Dysmenorrhoea - 35
- Ear infection - 36
- Fever - 37
- Flu - 38
- Gingivitis - 39
- Halitosis - 40
- Hay Fever - 41
- Headache - 42
- Heartburn - 43
- Hiccups - 44
- High blood pressure - 45
- Influenza - 46
- Insect bites - 48
- Insomnia - 49
- Laryngitis - 50
- Leg Cramps - 51
- Lumbago - 52
- Mouth ulcers - 53
- Neuralgia - 54
- Nose bleed - 55
- Sinusitis - 56
- Sore throat - 57

WAYS TO USE ESSENTIAL OIL - 63

SAFETY TIPS - 71

LIST OF CARRIER OILS - 75

- Almond
- Grape seed oil
- Avocado oil
- Olive oil
- Sesame oil
- Canola
- Sunflower oil
- Jojoba oil
- Emu oil
- Castor oil
- Borage seed oil
- Fractionated coconut oil

Other Books By Jack Pental

LEGAL NOTES

This Book contains information about treating medical ailments with essential oil. The information is not advice, and should not be treated as such.

[You must not rely on the information in this Book as an alternative to medical advice from an appropriately qualified professional. If you have any specific questions about any medical matter you should consult an appropriately qualified professional.]

[If you think you may be suffering from any medical condition you should seek immediate medical attention. You should never delay seeking medical advice, disregard medical advice, or discontinue medical treatment because of information in this Book.]

This Book is for informational purposes only.

AILMENTS

ABDOMINAL PAIN

Abdominal pain may be caused by digestive problems, cystitis, and menstruation, pulled muscles or simply eating too fast.

Drinking herbal teas made from mint or chamomile may help relieve some of the symptoms.

Massage oil may help and can be mixed as follows:

- 5 ml Carrier oil mixed with
- 1 drop Peppermint oil
- 1 drop of Chamomile
- 1 drop Clove oil

Mix together and gently massage the stomach area using a clockwise motion.

Medical advice should be sought if the pain persists accompanied by fever, headache, diarrhea and/or vomiting.

ABSCESS

An abscess typically is a pustular infection where the skin develops into a painful elevated lump.

Abscesses usually are eliminated though the surface of the skin in about two weeks, except in very rare circumstances.

To help ease the pain, make a compress using:

- 2 drops Chamomile essential oil
- 2 drops Lavender essential oil
- 2 drops Tea Tree essential oil

Apply twice a day to the swollen area.

ACNE

Mild acne is characterized by pimples as well as blackheads and is a common skin problem. However, severe cases can be extremely painful, causing enlarged pores.

Acne skin is very sensitive, so always clean the skin meticulously. Eat a well balanced diet and avoid fatty foods. Make sure to get plenty of exercise.

Essential oil can be applied neat to individual marks:

- Lavender oil
- Tea tree oil

Apply at night after cleaning, using clean cotton swab and continue until the acne spot has completely disappeared.

A facial treatment oil may also be used. Use suitable carrier oil, such as jojoba and add:

- Benzoin
- German chamomile
- Geranium
- Lavender
- Lemongrass
- Tea tree oil
- The inclusion of these essential oils listed for the facial treatment must **NOT EXCEED** a 2% dilution.

ATHLETE'S FOOT

Athlete's foot is a common fungal infection. Symptoms begin with small blisters that soon become inflamed patches that itch and burn.

The condition is highly contagious and flourishes in a damp moist environments.

Sweaty feet and poor hygiene can produce an environment for the fungus to grow in. Synthetic materials worn on the feet hinder the circulation of air and tend to promote dampness. This dampness makes for a favourable environment for the fungus to grow.

Prevention:

When going to a place where the infection might be contracted (such as public showers, pools ect.), rub the feet before and after with neat Geranium oil or Tea Tree oil.

Treatment:

To treat an infected foot mix:

- 10 ml of any carrier oil
- 2 drops Wheat germ oil
- 2 drops Tea Tree oil
- 2 drops Geranium oil

Rub in between the toes and around the nails every day.

BAD BREATH

Bad breath is a symptom of an underlying problem. Causes for bad breath can be anything from plaque build-up and decomposing food between the teeth to an infection.

Strong foods such as onions and garlic also add to bad breath. It may also be a sign of stomach problems, such as indigestion, or the improper elimination of toxins by the kidneys and the liver.

Mouth Wash:

- 125 ml warm water
- 5 ml Brandy
- 4 drops Lavender oil

Use this mixture by swishing and swirling around the mouth. Spit it out when finished. Do not swallow.

BEDSORES

Bedsores are places of ulceration, occurring on the body due to constant pressure and irritation.

These sores are usually on the heels, elbows and buttocks of bedridden people. Turning the person as often as possible can prevent the sores.

Massage oil to use both before and after sores develop:

- 20 ml carrier oil - such as Evening primrose oil
- 4 drops Wheat germ oil
- 3 drops Chamomile or Geranium oil
- 2 drops Lavender oil
- 2 drops Tea tree oil
- 2 drops Frankincense oil

Massage very gently into affected areas. Do not apply the massage oil if you are faced with a weeping bedsore...

BLEEDING

For small open wounds only. Apply a compress with the following added:

- 1 drop Lemon oil
- 1 drop Tea Tree oil
- 1 drop Chamomile oil
- 1 drop Geranium oil

BLEEDING GUMS

Bleeding gums are mostly caused by gingivitis which is an infection or inflammation of the gum. The irritation is mostly caused by plaque that lives in the mouth

To prepare a mouthwash:

1teaspoon of the following mixture to a glass of warm water:

- 3 drops of Peppermint oil
- 3 drops of Thyme oil
- 3 drops of Chamomile oil
- 2 drops of Eucalyptus oil
- Diluted in 1 tablespoon of brandy.

Swish and rinse the warm water with the 1 teaspoon of mixture around the mouth. Do not swallow.

If the problem continues, please contact your dentist immediately.

BLEPHARITIS

Blepharitis is an inflammation of the outer edge of the eyelid and is usually associated with bacterial (and sometimes viral) eye infection. It causes itching, burning and redness and sometimes a sensation of having something in one's eye. In addition to the irritation, there is sometimes a sticky matter in the eye that accompanies the infection.

Make a compress with the following:

- 30 ml Rosewater
- 5 ml Witch hazel
- 1 drop of Chamomile oil
- Mix well

Leave for at least 8 hours, then strain through a paper coffee filter. Take it and then use it as a compress on the closed eyelids.

BLISTERS

Blisters occur when there is an accumulation of fluid underneath the skin. When the blister bursts, the exposed tissue beneath may become infected.

Do not pierce blisters that are due to burns or scalds.

Apply:

- 1 drop Lavender oil or Tea tree oil, and
- 1 drop of Chamomile oil onto the blister.

Carefully pat it in.

BOILS

A boil is an abscess that may be located in such places as the buttocks, hairline or underarms. Swollen lymph glands, fever and fatigue may also be associated with boils.

Bathe the infected area with the combination of:

- 2 drops of Tea tree oil
- 2 drops Lavender oil
- 1drop Chamomile oil
- 1drop Juniper oil
- 200 ml hot water.

Bathe the infected area twice a day.

Please consult your medical practitioner if the condition worsens.

BRONCHITIS

This is an infection of the bronchial tubes and typically occurs with an existing cold and a dry, shallow cough. As phlegm develops the cough becomes painful.

The chest feels tight causing shortness of breath. Other symptoms may include aching muscles, chills, fever, sore throat and a runny nose.

Drink plenty of fluid, especially fresh lemon and pineapple juices and hot herbal teas.

Use inhalation therapy with the following essential oils:

- Pine
- Basil
- Benzoin
- Frankincense
- Clove
- Tea Tree oil

In addition to the inhalation therapy, vaporize the room during the day and one hour before bedtime with a mixture of 600 ml warm water, 15 drops Eucalyptus oil and 5 drops of Oregano oil.

BRUISING

A bruise develops when blood escapes from damaged blood vessels into the surrounding tissues under the skin.

Bruises may start out as black, blue or red skin and can change to a greenish yellow. Bruises may be caused by bumps, pinches and falls or when bones break.

If one suffers from anemia or obesity, the susceptibility of bruising increases. Adding dietary vitamin C may also help to prevent bruising and can speed the healing process.

Gently rub the affected area with the following massage oil:

- 10 ml Grape seed oil mixed with
- 5 drops Calendula oil
- 2 drops Fennel oil
- 1 drop Cypress oil

In addition to the massage oil, using neat Lavender oil may also be applied to the bruised area.

BURNS

For mild burns. Severe burns require immediate medical attention.

Immediately apply Lavender oil neat to the burn and cover with a damp compress.

CATARRH

Catarrh is the excessive secretion of phlegm from the air passage of the sinuses, larynx and lungs.

The causes of catarrh are colds, flu, hay fever, bronchitis, sinusitis, rhinitis and food allergies.

Mix in a bowl of hot water:

- Eucalyptus oil
- Thyme oil
- Place a towel over your head and breathe for 10 minutes.

Massage oil can also be rubbed on the chest and back area:

- 15 ml Evening primrose oil
- 3 drops Eucalyptus oil
- 3 drops Tea tree oil
- 3 drops Rosemary oil.

CHAPPED LIPS

To help ease the pain, and to assist in healing, apply oil mixture to lips:

- 20 ml Aloe vera oil
- 2 drops Rose oil
- 2 drops Geranium oil
- 1 drop Chamomile oil
- 1 drop Neroli oil

COLD SORES

A cold sore is a painful blisters around the lips. Typically it takes about ten days to heal. Once a crust has formed, the healing process has begun.

Cold sores are due to an outbreak of herpes simplex virus that can lay dormant for a long period of time.

Use Neat relieve the pain and swelling any of the following:

- Calendula oil
- Geranium oil
- Chamomile oil
- Tea tree oil

COLDS

The symptoms of a cold often are a stuffed-up runny nose, sneezing, and a sore throat.

Be sure to drink plenty of fluid when suffering from a cold, especially lemon water.

Safe Guard Spray for a room:

- 1 drop Pine essential oil
- 1 drop Eucalyptus essential oil
- 1 drop Cinnamon essential oil
- 1 drop Cloves essential oil
- 1 drop Niaouli essential oil

Mix the oils in 500 ml of water and place in a spray bottle. Shake well before use. Spray the room to be treated along with any surfaces that may be contaminated.

To relieve the stuffiness of a cold, use any combination of:

- Eucalyptus oil
- Pine oil
- Cloves oil
- Cajuput oil
- Niaouli oil

Sprinkle combination of oils on a handkerchief or use in an inhaler or in bath water. If using a chest rub, be sure to mix in suitable carrier oil.

CONJUNCTIVITIS

. Conjunctivitis is an infection of the outermost layer of the eye. It is also better known by the name, "Pink Eye".

This infection usually resolves itself in about ten days. Symptoms include redness, irritation, itching, burning and tearing.

Make a compress with the following:

- 1 drop of Chamomile oil
- 5 ml Witch hazel
- 30ml Rosewater

Mix well. Leave it for at least 7 hours, then strain through a paper coffee filter. Take the paper filter and use it as a compress on the closed eyelids.

CONSTIPATION

Constipation is the difficulty in passing stools, or the absence of an urge to eliminate waste and may be associated with bloating, mild nausea or indigestion.

Eat a diet rich in fiber-fresh fruit and vegetables. Avoid coffee, tea and chocolate. Exercise regularly.

Massage oil:

Apply clockwise over the lower abdomen three times a day:

- 30 ml jojoba oil
- 15 drops rosemary oil
- 10 drops lemon oil
- 5 drops peppermint oil

COUGHING

An irritation in the respiratory system usually causes a cough.

Use **steam inhalation** with:

- Eucalyptus oil

Use massage **oil**:

- 1 drop Pine oil
- 2 drops Thyme oil
- 3 drops Eucalyptus oil
- 1 teaspoon of Jojoba oil.

Use the above massage oil to massage the chest, back and neck...

Use a **mixture:**

- 2 drops Lemon oil
- 2 drops Eucalyptus oil
- 3 tablespoons honey

In a half a glass of warm water, use 1 teaspoon of the above combination and sip slowly.

DIARRHEA

Diarrhea is the bowels natural reaction to rid the body of unwanted substances.

Diarrhea may cause dehydration. Be sure to drink plenty of water and avoid foods such as fruit and dairy for a few days.

Massage oil may help ease the problem of diarrhea:

Make the massage oil; mix the essential oils to 10 ml vegetable carrier oil:

- 2 drops Eucalyptus oil
- 2 drops Peppermint oil
- 2 drops Chamomile oil
- 2 drops Lavender oil
- 2 drops Geranium oil
- 10 ml of vegetable carrier oil

Mix the essential oil with the carrier oil, and then rub over the abdomen.

DIVERTICULITIS

The diverticula of the weekend large intestine become inflamed and may cause tenderness, constipation, diarrhea, fever, spasms, anemia and bleeding.

Massage **oil** may ease the discomfort. In a clockwise motion, rub the oil over the stomach:

- 5 ml vegetable carrier oil.
- 1 drop Clove oil
- 1 drop Peppermint oil
- 1 drop Chamomile oil
- 2 drops Rosemary oil

DYSMENORRHOEA (PAINFUL MENSTRUATING)

Dysmenorrhoea can involve headaches, lower abdominal cramps and low back pain. Eat foods rich in magnesium and calcium. Such as nuts, seeds, dairy products and canned fish. These foods should be eaten before a period starts, as they are needed for muscle relaxation.

Massage oil may be used to help. Mix:

- 15 ml Jojoba oil
- 2 drops Geranium essential oil
- 2 drops Lavender essential oil
- 2 drops Bay essential oil
- 2 drops Clary sage essential oil
- 1 drop Peppermint essential oil

Massage externally over the painful area.

EAR INFECTION

Ear pain is usually caused by a middle-ear infection.

Symptoms may include a feeling of fullness in the ear, shooting pains in one or both ears, fever, and nausea, vomiting, and possibly hearing noises in the ear.

If the pain is very severe and there is neck stiffness and raised temperature, it is important to see a doctor.

For pain relief, mix:

1 drop Clove oil and 5 ml Grape seed oil and massage around the neck and ear.

FEVER

A fever is not a disease, but rather a mechanism of the body to combat infection. Fevers that get too high can cause seizures or even delirium which can affect the brain.

Drink plenty fluids like juice and mineral water to replace lost liquids during a fever episode.

Make massage oil and massage the temples, back of neck, top of hands and soles of feet.

Combine the following:

- 15 ml Evening primrose oil
- 2 drops Peppermint essential oil
- 2 drops Lavender essential oil
- 2 drops Eucalyptus essential oil
- 1 drop Tea Tree essential oil
- 1 drop Black pepper essential oil
- 1 drop Rosemary essential oil

FLU

Flu is much more severe than a cold, but tends to exhibit similar symptoms. Flu viruses are stronger, more infectious and harmful than those of colds. They are highly contagious. Drink plenty of fluids to replace losses due to fever. Stay in bed and rest.

At the first signs of flu, make a bath and add the following:

- 4 drops Tea tree oil
- 3 drops Lavender oil
- 1 drop Lemon oil

After the bath, apply massage oil:

- 10 ml Evening primrose oil
- 3 drops Tea tree oil
- 2 drops Eucalyptus oil

Use a vaporizer in the rooms you spend the most time in. Especially your bedroom when you sleep. Vaporize Pine, Lavender and Clove essential oils to help ease the flu symptoms.

GINGIVITIS

Gingivitis is an infection or inflammation of the gum, mostly in the tissue around the teeth.

To prepare a mouthwash to assist in fighting Gingivitis, do the following:

1 teaspoon of the following mixture to a glass of warm water:

- 3 drops of Peppermint oil
- 3 drops of Thyme oil
- 3 drops of Chamomile oil
- 2 drops of Eucalyptus oil
- Diluted the above in 1 tablespoon brandy.

Swish the warm water with the 1 teaspoon of mixture well around the mouth, but do NOT swallow.

If the problem persists, please consult your dentist immediately.

HALITOSIS

Bad breath is not a disease, but rather a symptom of an underlying problem. Causes of bad breath can be anything from decomposing food between the teeth, plaque build-up to improper digestion or improper removal of toxins from the body by the kidneys and liver.

For a mouthwash:

- 1 drop Myrrh oil to a cup of cooled, boiled water.

For a general mouthwash mix:

- 125 ml warm water.
- 5 ml brandy and
- 4 drops Lavender oil

Rinse the mixture around the mouth after proper brushing and flossing. Do not swallow.

HAY FEVER

Put a few drops:

- Eucalyptus oil
- Niaouli oil
- Tea Tree oil

    Place on a handkerchief and use it when an attack occurs.

HEADACHE

Massage into the base of the skull or around the temples:

- 3 drops Jojoba oil
- 3 drops Lavender oil
- 1 drop Bergamot oil
- 1 drop Peppermint oil

TENSION OR NERVOUS HEADACHE:

Massage into the base of the skull or around the temples:

- 3 drops of Lavender oil
- 2 drops Jojoba oil.
- 1 drop Clary sage oil
- 1 drop of Chamomile oil

HEARTBURN

Heartburn is a burning pain in the chest, which radiates upwards into throat and neck. It usually occurs after a meal when the stomach acids reflux up past the sphincter.

Rub the upper abdominal area with:

- 2 drops Eucalyptus oil
- 2 drops Fennel oil
- 1 drop Peppermint oil
- Diluted in 5ml (1 teaspoon) Grape seed oil.

HICCUPS

Place 1 drop :

- Chamomile oil

    In a brown paper bag and hold over your nose and mouth. Breathe in slowly and deeply through your nose.

HIGH BLOOD PRESSURE

Hypertension or high blood pressure occurs when excessive force is exerted against the artery wall as the heart pumps blood. If left uncontrolled, high blood pressure can lead to stroke, kidney failure or a heart attack.

*** ESSENTIAL OILS TO BE **AVOIDED** FOR USE WITH HIGH BLOOD PRESSURE

- Thyme (hypertensive - increase blood pressure)
- Hyssop (contains pinocamphone)
- Sage (contains thujone)
- Rosemary (very stimulating)

ESSENTIAL OILS THAT MAY BE **BENEFICIAL** IN MASSAGE FOR PEOPLE SUFFERING FROM HIGH BLOOD PRESSURE:

- Ylang-ylang
- Clary sage
- Lavender
- Melissa
- Marjoram

INFLUENZA

The flu is an infection caused by a virus. The symptoms may include aching muscles, headache, fever, chest pains, sore throat, coughing and sweating.

Be sure to drink plenty of liquids to rehydrate, especially if there is a fever.

To help protect your home against influenza:

- 1 drop Pine essential oil
- 1 drop Cinnamon essential oil
- 1 drop Cloves essential oil
- 1 drop Eucalyptus essential oil
- 1 drop Niaouli essential oil

Mix the oils in 500 ml water and put in a spray bottle. After shaking, spray the rooms that you wish to protect.

To remove the 'stuffed up' feeling of flu symptoms, use any combination of:

- Pine
- Eucalyptus
- Cloves
- Cajuput
- Niaouli

Use in a bath or by an inhalation method. If using as a chest rub, be sure to use carrier oil such as Jojoba oil.

INSECT BITES

Remove the sting by applying the neat essential oil onto the site.

As an insect repellant use:

- Lavender oil
- Lemongrass oil
- Citronella oil (especially effective for mosquitoes)
- Thyme oil
- Peppermint oil

INSOMNIA

Insomnia means that one is unable to sleep.

Take a warm bath using:

- Lavender oil
- Neroli oil

    Place a few drops of each oil in a warm bath half an hour before bedtime to help relax.

As a relaxing massage, use any combination:

- Lavender oil
- Clary sage oil
- Petitgrain oil
- Sandalwood oil
- Ylang ylang oil

Mix in suitable carrier oil.

LARYNGITIS

Laryngitis is an inflammation of the larynx, which interferes with speech. In more serious cases, a person may have no voice at all and breathing and swallowing can be very difficult.

For a sore throat gargle five to six times a day with a glass of cooled boiled water and 2 drops of either:

- Black Pepper
- Rosemary
- Cajuput
- Tea Tree
- Geranium
- Niaouli

Steam inhalation add:

- 2 drops Lavender
- 1 drop Eucalyptus
- 1 drop Thyme
- 1 drop Chamomile

LEG CRAMPS

Cramp is the sudden involuntary contraction of a muscle or group of muscles, and can cause acute pain.

Consult your doctor if the cramps are very severe.

As a massage, rub the legs vigorously with the following mixture until the cramp is relieved.

- 3 drops of Geranium essential oil
- 5 ml Evening primrose oil

  .Cramps may also be relieved by bending the knee as far as possible.

LUMBAGO

Lumbago is a severe pain in the lumbar region of the spine, (the lower back).

Bed rest, heat and massage are ways to relieve the pain and the pressure. Stay in bed for a few days with a large cushion under the knees to rest the back.

Hot Bath add 3 drops total of either:

- Thyme oil
- Rosemary oil
- or Oregano

Massage oil:

Massage with the oil mixture the lower back down to the top end of buttocks. Avoid the anus since the oils may cause irritation.

Mix the following oils together:

- 10 ml Evening primrose oil
- 3 drops Rosemary oil
- 2 drops Chamomile oil
- 2 drops Peppermint oil
- 1 drop Eucalyptus oil
- 1 drop Cardamom oil

MOUTH ULCERS

Aphthous ulcers are tiny open sores which develop in the mouth, on the tongue, the roof of the mouth, on the mucus membrane inside the lips and cheeks. Ulcers can last from two days to three weeks.

A cotton ball dipped in Tea Tree oil may be applied neat to the ulcer for the immediate relief of soreness.

As a mouthwash use:

- 5ml salt
- 2 drops of Tea Tree oil
- 500 ml warm boiled water.

Another mouthwash:

- 1 glass of warm water
- 10 ml brandy
- 2 drops Tea tree oil
- 2 drops Peppermint oil
- 2 drops Thyme oil
- 2 drops Geranium oil
- 2 drops Lemon oil

Swish mouth wash around mouth. Do not swallow.

NEURALGIA

When a nerve is irritated, inflamed or compressed, pain is felt. Any inflammation or infection can cause it.

Massage oil may assist with neuralgia:

- 10 ml Grape seed oil
- 3 drops Lavender oil
- 3 drops Black Pepper oil
- 3 drops Chamomile oil
- 1 drop Clove oil

NOSE BLEED

For a nosebleed that is not due to an injury, pinch the nostrils and inhale the following oils from a tissue:

- 1 drop Lavender oil
- 3 drops Lemon oil

An icepack may also be applied.

For a nosebleed due to an injury, see your doctor immediately.

SINUSITIS

Sinusitis is a bacterial infection or inflammation of one or more of the sinus passages located in the bones surrounding the eyes and nose.

Use steam inhalation for relief of the pain with the following essential oils added:

- 1 drop Thyme oil
- 1 drop Eucalyptus oil
- 2 drops Rosemary oil
- 2 drops Peppermint oil

Use massage oil after the inhalation:

- 10 ml suitable carrier oil
- 3 drops Rosemary oil
- 3 drops Geranium oil
- 2 drops Eucalyptus oil
- 2 drops Peppermint oil
- 1 drop Tea tree oil

SORE THROAT

Sore throat or pharyngitis usually indicates inflammation of the pharynx, which extends from the back of the mouth to the esophagus. Common types of sore throat are viral and bacterial infection and tonsillitis.

To alleviate discomfort, massage oil can be applied to the back of the ears and neck:

- 5 ml vegetable carrier oil.
- 4 drops Chamomile essential oil
- 1 drop Tea tree essential oil
- 1 drop Thyme essential oil
- 1 drop Lemon essential oil

Steam inhalation may also be helpful:

- 2 drops Lavender

- 2 drops Eucalyptus

- 1 drop Thyme oil

Use a humidifier to keep the air moist. Drink plenty of fluids.

SWOLLEN ANKLES

Ankles can swell for many reasons. Resting with the feet up is always an effective cure.

Drink plenty of fluid and massage from the feet up to the knees with the following:

- 30 ml Evening primrose oil.
- 15 drops Cypress oil
- 15 drops Fennel oil

TOOTHACHE

Put a drop of clove oil on a cotton ball and apply it to the gum around the tooth or into the crevices on either side.

The cheek and jawbone may also be massaged:

- 5 ml vegetable oil.
- 3 drops Chamomile oil
- 1 drop Clove oil
- 1 drop Lemon oil

VARICOSE VEINS

Varicose veins are most common in the legs; however they can occur in various parts of the body. .

For some pain relief, gently massage the legs daily, working up the legs from the feet towards the heart:

- 20 ml Almond oil
- 4 drops Lavender oil
- 4 drops Cypress oil
- 2 drops Wheat germ oil

WOUNDS

Bathe the area with 500 ml warm water with the following essential oils added:

- 2 drops Tea Tree oil
- 5 drops Lavender oil

When covering up the wound, put 3 drops Lavender oil on a piece of gauze and place it over the cut.

Repeat twice a day for two days. On the third day, expose the wound to air.

If there is any doubt of the seriousness of the wound, please visit your emergency room.

WAYS TO USE ESSENTIAL OIL

There are many ways in which essential oils may be used. The ones listed in this book are:

- Air freshening
- Bathing
- Compresses
- Massage
- Steam inhalations
- Vaporization / diffusing

Even though the use of essential oils is beneficial to a person's health, one must remember that they are very concentrated and safety must always be adhered to.

AIR FRESHENING

- Take a clean plastic spray bottle (used for spraying plants) and half fill it with clean water.
- Add 8 - 10 drops of your desired essential oil to the water and shake well.
- Shake the bottle and give the room a couple of quick sprays. Make sure not to spray near polished furniture, as the essential oils can damage the polished surface.
- When not using, store the bottle in a dark cool area.

BATHING

You would normally add about 7 drops of essential oils to a bath, but if you have a sensitive skin, or it's the first time trying a new oil, first mix the essential oil to a carrier oil or a small amount of shampoo and then add it to your bath.

- Add the oils after you have run the bath, and then to mix in by hand.

- Children ages 4 to 12, as well as for elderly people, only add 4 drops of oil per bath.

- For children ages 1 to 4, as well as for pregnant women, add only 2 drops of oil per bath.

- Children under 1 year should have no more than 1 drop of oil per bath.

COMPRESSES

To make a **hot compress**:

- Add about 4 drops of your selected essential oil to about a pint of hot water.
- Then place your folded piece of material on top of the water and let it soak it up.
- Next wring out the excess water and place it over the area to be treated.
- Cover the warm compress with a plastic bag or plastic wrap and another towel on top to keep it in place.
- Leave on, and replace with a new compress as soon as it has cooled to body temperature.

To make a **Cold compress**:

- A cold compress is made exactly the same as the hot compress, but ice or cold water is used instead of the hot water.
- The compress is replaced when it has heated up to body temperature.

MASSAGE

When you use essential oils for a massage, you will need to dilute with a suitable carrier oil, since essential oils are too concentrated to use undiluted on the skin.

Age	Amount of carrier oil	Amount of essential oil
65 years +	20 ml	5 drops
12 - 65	20 ml	10 drops
6 - 12	20 ml	7 drops
4 - 6	20 ml	5 drops
1 - 4	20 ml	2 drop
under 1	20 ml	1 drop
Pregnant	20 ml	1 drop

STEAM INHALATION

- Pour hot water into a bowl.
- Add 3 drops of the chosen essential oil.
- Place your head about 12 inches above the bowl and cover your head with a towel in such a way that the sides are totally closed, forming a tent above the bowl.
- Keep your eyes shut and breathe deeply through your nose for 1 to 2 minutes.

* If at any time you begin to feel uncomfortable, discontinue the treatment.

*When using this treatment with children or elderly people make sure that they do not burn themselves by getting too close to the bowl or spilling the hot water.

VAPORIZATION

- Depending on the size of the room, a good rule of thumb is to place about 5 - 8 drops of the essential oil to the water that is located in the reservoir on top.
- As the water heats up from the candle, the essential oil in the water will begin to evaporate, dispensing the aroma throughout the room.

Using an ultrasonic type of diffuser can be an alternative to the candle type of diffuser.

Rings that are placed on light bulbs can also be used. The oils are placed on the ring, and the ring is then placed on a turned off light bulb. As the bulb is heated up, the oil starts to dissipate.

SAFETY TIPS

Following these safety tips will help keep you safe while
using essential oils.

- Always dilute essential oils with suitable carrier oil
  before applying it to the skin.
- Never ingest or use essential oils internally.
- Always keep essential oils away from the reach of
  any children.
- Be careful not to get any essential oils on any
  mucous membranes or into your eyes.
- Always wash your hands after handling pure
  undiluted essential oils.
- If you have any medical condition or are pregnant,
  consult your aroma therapist or a doctor before
  using any essential oils.
- Some oils are not safe for use while pregnant. They
  have the possibility of causing contractions and
  premature delivery.
- Use essential oils with great care on children.
- If you are using a new un-tried essential oil, first do
  a skin patch test.
- If irritation occurs with a specific oil or formula,
  discontinue using it.
- Do not drink alcohol while using essential oils.

- Essential oils may interfere with certain medications. Check with your pharmacist or doctor for the possibility of any interaction before using essential oils.
- Essential oils may transfer through the skin to nursing babies. Essential oil selection must be carefully chosen if nursing.
- Avoid exposure to the sun while using oils that cause sensitivity to sunlight.
- Always perform a skin patch test before using any essential oil for the first time.

SKIN PATCH TEST

It is strongly recommended that you perform a skin patch test before using any essential oils for the first time, especially if you have a problem with sensitive skin.

Mix:

- 1 drop of the oil you wish to test
- 1 teaspoon (5 ml) of carrier oil - such as almond oil or sweet grape seed oil.
- Apply a small amount of the mixed oil to the inside of your elbow or wrist and leave uncovered for twenty four hours.
- Do not wash the area for this period of time.
- If no sign of itching, redness or swelling occurs after the 24 hour period, it should be safe for you to use the oil.

LIST OF COMMON CARRIER OILS

*Sweet almond oil and grape seed oil are very popular carrier oils.

Apricot Oil

- Apricot oil or apricot kernel oil is pressed from the kernels of the *Prunus armeniaca* (apricot)

Almond

- The oil is good for application to the skin as an emollient, and has been traditionally used by massage therapists to lubricate the skin during a massage session

Grape seed oil

- Light and thin, grape seed oil leaves a glossy film over skin when used as carrier oil for essential oils in aromatherapy. It contains more linoleic acid than many other carrier oils.

Avocado oil

- Avocado oil was originally, and still is, extracted for cosmetic use because of its very high skin penetration and rapid absorption.

Olive oil

- In ancient Greece, the substance was used during massage, to prevent sports injuries, relieve muscle fatigue, and eliminate lactic acid buildup.

Sesame oil

- In Ayurvedic medicine, sesame oil (til tel) is used for massaging as it is believed to rid the body of heat due to its viscous nature upon rubbing. It is also used for hair and scalp massage. It is also used in many cosmetic applications.

Canola

- Canola oil is low in saturated fat and contains both omega-6 and omega-3 fatty acids in a ratio of 2:1.

Sunflower oil

- In cosmetics, it has smoothing properties and is considered noncomedogenic.

Jojoba oil

- Jojoba oil is found as an additive in many cosmetic products, especially those marketed as being made from natural ingredients.

Emu oil

- Emu oil is oil derived from adipose tissue harvested from certain subspecies of the emu, *Dromaius novaehollandiae*, a flightless bird indigenous to Australia.

Castor oil

- Castor oil is well known as a source of ricinoleic acid, a monounsaturated, 18-carbon fatty acid.

Borage seed oil

- In herbal medicine, borage seed oil has been used for skin disorders such as eczema, seborrheic dermatitis, and neurodermatitis.

Fractionated coconut oil

- Coconut oil can be used as a skin moisturizer, helping with dry skin.

ABOUT THE AUTHOR

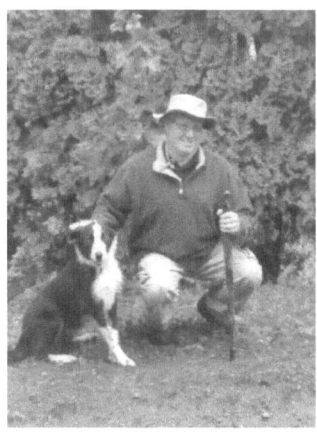

Jack is a former New York State Correctional Officer turned author. Jack draws upon his life experiences as an officer, husband, father and Christian to write books that attract a diverse audience. Jack lives in Upstate NY, in the foothills of the Adirondack Park, where he enjoys hiking, hunting and gardening. He shares his home with his wife, three children and faithful dog, Conan.

OTHER BOOKS BY JACK PENTAL

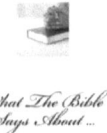

What The Bible Says About ...

Jack Pental   What the Bible Says About… (A Quick Reference Guide)- • **ISBN-10:** 1507757778 • **ISBN-13:** 978-1507757772